AYURVEDIC MASSAGE FOR BEGINNERS

Discover Healing Techniques, Stress Relief Methods, And Ancient Wellness Practices For Holistic Health And Relaxation

DR SAWYER DIEGO

Copyright © [2024] by [Dr. .Sawyer Diego]. All rights reserved.

Except for brief quotations included in critical reviews and certain other noncommercial uses allowed by copyright law, no part of this publication may be reproduced, distributed, or transmitted in any form or by any means, including photocopying, recording, or other electronic or mechanical methods, without the publisher's prior written permission.

DISCLAMER

Nothing in this book should be interpreted as medical advice; it is meant exclusively for educational reasons. Regarding their specific health issues and treatment options, readers are urged to speak with licensed healthcare professionals. The publisher and author disclaim all liability for any errors or omissions in the material provided, as well as for any negative effects that may arise from using or abusing the information. Although every attempt has been taken to guarantee that the material in this book is correct as of the date of publishing, new research may have superseded some of the content because medical knowledge is always changing. It is recommended that readers confirm the most recent medical recommendations and guidelines. The reader of this book undertakes to release the author and publisher from any claims or liabilities resulting from the use of this information, and understands and accepts the inherent risks connected with healthcare decisions.

TABLE OF CONTENTS

CHAPTER ONE 11
  AYURVEDIC MASSAGE OVERVIEW 11
    AYURVEDIC MASSAGE: WHAT IS IT? 11
    AYURVEDIC MASSAGE BENEFITS 13
    COMPREHENDING AYURVEDIC DOSHAS 14
    THE VALUE OF HARMONY IN HEALTH 16

CHAPTER TWO 19
  THE BASIS OF AYURVEDA 19
    AYURVEDIC PHILOSOPHY AND HISTORY 19
    THE FUNDAMENTALS OF AYURVEDIC MEDICINE 21
    AN OVERVIEW OF THE DOSHAS (AYURVEDIC BODY TYPES) ... 23
    THE LIFE FORCE, OR PRANA, CONCEPT 24
    MASSAGE'S FUNCTION IN AYURVEDA 26

CHAPTER THREE 29
  HOW TO BEGIN RECEIVING AYURVEDIC MASSAGE 29
    SETTING UP YOUR AREA AND YOURSELF 29
    ESSENTIAL BASIC EQUIPMENT 30
    THE ENVIRONMENT IS IMPORTANT FOR MASSAGE 32
    HYGIENE AND SAFETY PROCEDURES 33
    ESTABLISHING GOALS FOR THE MASSAGE 35

CHAPTER FOUR 37
  THE APPLICATIONS OF AYURVEDIC OILS 37
    A SUMMARY OF VITAL AYURVEDIC OILS 37
    QUALITIES AND ADVANTAGES OF ESSENTIAL OILS 38

- COMBINING OILS FOR VARIOUS DOSHAS 40
- SELECTING THE PROPER OIL BASED ON YOUR BODY TYPE 41
- TECHNIQUES FOR USING OIL IN MASSAGE 43

CHAPTER FIVE 45
- AYURVEDIC MASSAGE METHODS 45
  - ABHYANGA: CONVENTIONAL METHOD OF SELF-MASSAGE 45
  - VARIOUS STROKES AND THEIR OBJECTIVES 46
  - IN AN AYURVEDIC MASSAGE, MARMA POINTS 47
  - CHANGING PRESSURE BASED ON DOSHA 48
  - INCLUDING AWARENESS OF BREATH 49

CHAPTER SIX 51
- AYURVEDIC MASSAGE BENEFITS 51
  - PHYSICAL ADVANTAGES: CIRCULATION, MUSCLE RELAXATION, AND JOINT HEALTH 51
  - BENEFITS FOR THE MIND: REDUCTION OF STRESS AND 52
  - EFFECTS OF DETOXIFICATION AND CLEANING 53
  - BOOSTING VITALITY AND IMMUNITY 54
  - BENEFITS OF REGULAR PRACTICE OVER TIME 55

CHAPTER SEVEN 57
- TAILORING YOUR PRACTICE TO AYURVEDIC MASSAGE 57
  - MASSAGING DEPENDING ON THE SEASON (RITUCHARYA) 57
  - MODIFYING METHODS CONSIDERING AGE AND 58
  - TAKING CARE OF PARTICULAR HEALTH ISSUES 60
  - INCLUDING AYURVEDIC PRINCIPLES IN EVERYDAY LIVING 61
  - MASSAGE TECHNIQUES FOR FAMILIES AND PARTNERS 63

CHAPTER EIGHT 65
AYURVEDIC PRACTICES FOR SELF-CARE 65
DAILY ROUTINES FOR AYURVEDIC SELF-CARE 65
ROUTINES ARE IMPORTANT (DINACHARYA) 67
AYURVEDIC FOOD RECOMMENDATIONS FOR OPTIMAL 68
USING SPICES AND HERBS TO MAINTAIN BALANCE 70
MASSAGE IN CONJUNCTION WITH YOGA AND MEDITATION 71

CHAPTER NINE 73
FAQS & FREQUENTLY ASKED QUESTIONS 73
INTOLERANCES AND HYPERSENSITIVITY TO OILS 73
PRECAUTIONARY MEASURES FOR EXPECTANT MOTHERS 75
MODIFYING MASSAGE FOR OLDER OR ILL PEOPLE 76
RESOLVING DOUBT REGARDING AYURVEDIC METHODS 78
HOW OFTEN IS AN AYURVEDIC MASSAGE RECOMMENDED? 79

CHAPTER TEN 81
IMPROVING YOUR WORK 81
ADVANCED AYURVEDIC METHODS AND TREATMENTS 81
RESOURCES AND ONGOING EDUCATION 82
LOCATING ELIGIBLE AYURVEDIC PHYSICIANS 84
INCLUDING THE PHILOSOPHY OF AYURVEDA IN DAILY LIFE 86
EXAMINING WORKSHOPS & RETREATS FOR AYURVEDIC 88

CHAPTER ELEVEN 91
UPCOMING DEVELOPMENTS IN AYURVEDIC MASSAGE 91
CONTEMPORARY USES AND INNOVATIONS 91
GROWING WORLDWIDE ADOPTION OF AYURVEDIC PRACTICES 92

INTEGRATIVE METHODS IN MEDICAL PRACTICE 94

INVESTIGATIONS AND ADVANCEMENTS IN AYURVEDIC 96

NEW PROSPECTS FOR AYURVEDIC PROFESSIONALS 97

ABOUT THE BOOK

With a focus on the therapeutic art of massage, "Ayurvedic Massage for Beginners" offers a thorough introduction to the ancient healing tradition of Ayurveda. Based on centuries-old wisdom, Ayurveda emphasizes a holistic approach to wellness, seeing health as a harmonious balance between mind, body, and spirit. This book explores the philosophical underpinnings, rich history, and core idea of doshas, which are unique body types that determine temperament and health.

Ayurvedic massage, or Abhyanga, is a vital part of maintaining prana's balance within the body, which promotes overall well-being and longevity. The belief in prana, the vital life force that flows through all living beings, is central to Ayurvedic philosophy. This book provides readers with the knowledge they need to confidently begin their Ayurvedic massage journey through thorough explanations and practical guidance.

The book goes into great detail on practical matters like getting ready and setting up a massage room, including basic safety and hygiene measures. Readers will discover the significance of choosing oils based on their dosha type, investigating different qualities, and mixing methods to improve therapeutic effects. The book also explains individual massage techniques and marma points, which are important energy centers in the body, providing information on how to adjust pressure and use breath awareness for the best outcomes.

Beyond mere physical relaxation, Ayurvedic massages offers mental clarity, emotional balance, and stress relief. Regular application of the practice aids in detoxification increases immunity, and promotes vitality. Seasonally appropriate and individually tailored massage techniques (ritucharya) guarantee year-round holistic health benefits.

A thorough understanding and safe application of Ayurvedic massage techniques are ensured by answering common questions and concerns, including safety precautions for sensitive groups and adapting practices for varying health conditions. Furthermore, this guide emphasizes the integration of Ayurvedic principles into daily life through self-care rituals, dietary guidelines, and complementary practices like yoga and meditation.

The book delves into sophisticated treatments, contemporary uses, and developing patterns in Ayurvedic massage, mirroring the practice's expanding worldwide appeal and assimilation into contemporary medical procedures. It offers resources for additional learning and locating certified practitioners, enabling Ayurvedic wellness to become attainable for individuals looking for deep recovery and wholeness in their lives.

CHAPTER ONE
AYURVEDIC MASSAGE OVERVIEW
AYURVEDIC MASSAGE: WHAT IS IT?

Deeply ingrained in ancient Indian healing traditions, Ayurvedic massage is a holistic therapy that seeks to balance the body, mind, and spirit. It goes beyond simple physical relaxation to balance the entire being. The core of Ayurvedic philosophy is the belief that every individual is composed of a distinct combination of the five elements (earth, water, fire, air, and ether), which manifest as three doshas (Vata, Pitta, and Kapha) that govern different physiological and psychological functions in the body. Consequently, Ayurvedic massage is customized based on the dosha constitution and particular health requirements of each client.

Ayurvedic massage, or "Abhyanga," involves the selection and heating of therapeutic oils to a comfortable temperature; the choice of oil is based on the season and the predominant dosha of the individual. The massage therapist applies the warm oil in gentle, rhythmic strokes, which help to lubricate the tissues, improve circulation, and relax the muscles. The strokes follow the direction of the body's natural energy flow, promoting the release of toxins and enhancing overall vitality. Typically, the massage concentrates on marma points, which are vital energy centers believed to be the concentrated sites of the body's life force. This holistic approach seeks to rejuvenate the body while also calming the mind and restoring emotional balance.

Understanding the principles and techniques of Ayurvedic massage allows individuals to embark on a journey of self-care and holistic health, aligning with the ancient wisdom that views each person as a unique embodiment of the elements and energies of the universe. Regular practice of Ayurvedic massage is believed to prevent illness by maintaining the balance of the doshas and supporting the body's natural healing processes.

Ayurvedic massage is not merely a physical treatment but a deeply therapeutic experience that nurtures both the body and the spirit.

AYURVEDIC MASSAGE BENEFITS

The physical, mental, and emotional well-being benefits of Ayurvedic massage go far beyond relaxation. It helps with blood circulation, lymphatic drainage, and toxin removal from the body. It also relieves tension and stiffness in the muscles, improves joint mobility, and supports overall flexibility.

The therapeutic oils used in Ayurvedic massage penetrate deeply into the skin, nourishing tissues and supporting healthy skin tone.

Anxiety and depression can be reduced, improving mental clarity and emotional stability. Regular sessions can alleviate depression and anxiety. By balancing the doshas, Ayurvedic massage harmonizes the mind-body connection, fostering a sense of inner peace and emotional resilience. Deep relaxation and tranquility are instilled on a mental and emotional level by the rhythmic strokes and gentle pressure.

Beyond its physical and psychological benefits, Ayurvedic massage encourages self-awareness and mindfulness, nurturing a deeper understanding of one's unique constitution and health needs. As a holistic therapy, it empowers individuals to take an active role in their well-being, promoting a balanced and harmonious lifestyle in tune with nature's rhythms. Beyond its benefits to the body, Ayurvedic massage also plays a crucial role in preventive healthcare by strengthening the immune system and enhancing overall vitality.

COMPREHENDING AYURVEDIC DOSHAS

According to Ayurveda, the three basic energies known as doshas—Vata, Pitta, and Kapha—are responsible for all bodily functions that are biological, psychological, and emotional. Each dosha is a blend of the five elements—earth, water, fire, air, and ether—and each one expresses itself differently in each individual. Vata, which is made up of air and ether, regulates movement and communication in the body and is linked to characteristics like dryness, lightness, and creativity. Pitta, which is composed of fire and water, controls metabolism and transformation and is linked to heat, intensity, and determination. Finally, Pitta, composed of earth and water, regulates structure and cohesiveness and is linked to characteristics like stability, heaviness, and nurturing.

Ayurvedic principles emphasize the importance of maintaining harmony among the doshas to achieve optimal health and well-being. Individualized lifestyle choices, such as diet, exercise, and daily routines, are tailored to balance the predominant doshas and prevent illness. By aligning with the natural rhythms of the body and the environment, people can support their innate constitution and promote longevity and vitality. Knowledge of the doshas helps people recognize their unique constitution, known as

Prakriti, and understand how imbalances can manifest as physical or emotional symptoms.

Ayurvedic therapies, such as diet modifications, herbal remedies, yoga, meditation, and massage, are designed to restore balance and harmony to the doshas. Ayurveda promotes holistic healing and empowers individuals to cultivate health and vitality from within by addressing the underlying cause of imbalance. Embracing the wisdom of the doshas allows individuals to live in harmony with their natural constitution and achieve a state of equilibrium that supports overall well-being. The doshas are not static; they fluctuate according to various factors, including diet, stress, environment, and seasonal changes.

THE VALUE OF HARMONY IN HEALTH

Ayurveda views health holistically, taking into account not only physical symptoms but also mental and emotional states. Balance is upheld by being aware of one's constitution, or Prakriti, and comprehending the interplay of the doshas—Vata, Pitta, and Kapha. In Ayurveda, optimal well-being is achieved through harmony among the body, mind, and spirit. The concept of balance extends beyond the absence of disease to encompass a dynamic state of equilibrium that supports vitality and resilience.

To keep the doshas in balance, one must nurture them according to their inherent tendencies and qualities. For example, Vata, the mind-body mind, responds best to grounding practices like regular routines, nourishing foods, and warm, calming therapies; Pitta, the mind-body transformation and metabolism, responds best to cooling foods, relaxation techniques, and activities that encourage emotional cooling; and Kapha, the mind-body structure and cohesion, responds best to stimulating practices like vigorous exercise, light foods, and energizing therapies.

Ayurvedic practices such as yoga, meditation, and therapeutic massage reflect the importance of balance in health; they promote harmony among the doshas and support overall well-being. By cultivating awareness of their unique constitution and making informed lifestyle choices, individuals can sustain optimal health and vitality throughout their lives. Ayurvedic lifestyles recommendations, including diet, exercise, sleep patterns, and stress management, are tailored to individual constitutions and seasonal variations.

Ayurveda provides useful tools and principles to help people maintain equilibrium and prevent disease. People who embrace Ayurveda's wisdom can cultivate resilience, enhance vitality, and experience a profound sense of well-being. Maintaining balance in health requires a holistic approach that takes into account the interconnectedness of body, mind, and spirit. Balancing the doshas and nurturing health through personalized practices empowers people to take an active role in their wellness journey, promoting a harmonious and fulfilling life through natural rhythms and innate wisdom.

CHAPTER TWO
THE BASIS OF AYURVEDA
AYURVEDIC PHILOSOPHY AND HISTORY

The word "Ayurveda" itself translates to "the science of life" (Ayur = life, Veda = science or knowledge) and embodies a comprehensive approach to health and wellness. At the heart of Ayurvedic philosophy is the belief that health is a delicate balance between the body, mind, spirit, and environment.

This balance is influenced by various factors, including diet, lifestyle, emotions, and relationships. Ayurveda is a holistic medical system with a rich history and profound philosophy that dates back over 5,000 years, making it one of the oldest healing systems in the world.

Ayurveda is a holistic medicine that emphasizes disease prevention through appropriate diet, lifestyle choices, and therapies that support balance in the body and mind.

Its philosophy holds that each individual is a unique combination of the five elements found in the universe: space, air, fire, water, and earth. These elements combine to form three primary life energies or doshas: Vata (space and air), Pitta (fire and water), and Kapha (water and earth).

Ayurvedic knowledge grew over centuries and was organized into texts like the Charaka Samhita and Sushruta Samhita, which detail principles of diagnosis, treatment, and ethical medical conduct. Today, Ayurveda thrives as a comprehensive system of natural healing, integrating herbal remedies, dietary advice, yoga, meditation, and therapeutic practices to promote overall well-being. Ayurveda's historical development saw it evolve from ancient texts known as the Vedas, particularly the Atharva Veda, which contains early references to medical practices and herbal treatments.

THE FUNDAMENTALS OF AYURVEDIC MEDICINE

The fundamental tenets of Ayurvedic medicine inform both its diagnostic and therapeutic approaches. Vata, Pitta, and Kapha are the three doshas that control physiological functions; the balance of these doshas is essential to health. Vata, which is made up of elements of air and space, governs movement and is associated with activities like breathing and circulation.

Pitta, which is formed by fire and water, governs metabolism and digestion. Kapha, which is formed by water and earth, governs structure and stability in the body.

Ayurveda emphasizes the importance of strong Agni for overall health; digestive imbalances are seen as contributing factors to disease, and Ayurvedic treatments often aim to strengthen Agni through dietary adjustments, herbal remedies, and lifestyle modifications.

Another fundamental principle is the concept of Agni, or digestive fire, which is essential for processing nutrients and maintaining vitality.

Ayurvedic therapies incorporate practices that support mental clarity, emotional balance, and spiritual growth alongside physical healing because they acknowledge the interconnectedness of the mind and body, the importance of emotional well-being to physical health, and the possibility that mental disturbances may be the cause of illness.

Ayurvedic diagnosis entails evaluating these factors through detailed observation, pulse reading (Nadi Pariksha), and questioning to understand a person's unique constitution and current state of health. Treatment plans then focus on restoring balance through customized dietary recommendations, herbal formulas, detoxification therapies, and rejuvenating practices. Activities like meditation, yoga, and targeted herbal treatments are tailored to individual constitutions (Prakriti) and imbalances (Vikriti).

AN OVERVIEW OF THE DOSHAS (AYURVEDIC BODY TYPES)

Knowing one's body type, or dosha constitution, is essential to personalized health care in Ayurveda. The three doshas (Vata, Pitta, and Kapha) govern individual traits, inclinations toward imbalance, and suitable therapeutic approaches. Vata types are often vivacious, creative, and prone to anxiety when their dosha is out of balance; Pitta types are frequently intense, ambitious, and prone to problems like inflammation and heartburn; and Kapha types are usually calm, nurturing, and may gain weight and become lethargic when their dosha is disturbed.

Knowing one's predominant dosha helps customize diet, exercise, and daily routines to maintain or restore balance. For example, Vata types benefit from warm, grounding foods and routines that promote stability and relaxation; Pitta types thrive on cooling, calming activities and foods that support digestion without overheating; and Kapha types benefit from stimulating, invigorating practices that prevent stagnation and promote vitality. Each person's dosha composition is unique and influenced by genetics, environment, and lifestyle choices.

Ayurvedic practitioners evaluate doshas by physical examination, questioning, and pulse diagnosis to prescribe treatments that address specific imbalances. By aligning with one's natural constitution and making lifestyle adjustments accordingly, people can improve their general well-being and prevent disease. Dosha balance encompasses not only physical traits but also mental and emotional tendencies.

THE LIFE FORCE, OR PRANA, CONCEPT

The fundamental idea of Ayurveda is Prana, the life force that animates all living things. Prana is energy, vitality, and consciousness that permeates every cell and directs physiological processes. It flows through subtle channels called nadis and is affected by breath (Pranayama), food, thoughts, and emotions. According to Ayurvedic philosophy, maintaining a balanced Prana is necessary for long life and good health.

The doshas and their functions are closely related to Prana. Vata dosha, meaning movement, is connected to Prana flow throughout the body. Pitta dosha, meaning transformation and metabolism, determines how Prana is used for digestion and the production of cellular energy. Kapha dosha, meaning structure and stability, aids in the grounding and preservation of Prana within the body.

To maintain vitality, mental clarity, and emotional balance, Ayurvedic practices like yoga, pranayama (breath control), and meditation work to enhance Prana flow, clear blockages in the nadis, and harmonize the doshas.

Because optimal Prana circulation throughout the body is ensured, imbalances in Prana can manifest as physical ailments, fatigue, mental fog, or emotional disturbances, which is why Ayurvedic treatments aim to restore equilibrium and rejuvenate the life force.

Techniques for stimulating Prana flow, releasing tension, and promoting general wellness are used in Ayurvedic massage. This holistic approach recognizes the connection between Prana and all aspects of health; therefore it targets not just physical discomfort but also mental and emotional balance.

MASSAGE'S FUNCTION IN AYURVEDA

Ayurvedic massage, also referred to as Abhyanga, is an important part of Ayurvedic healing practices. It is a form of therapeutic and preventive medicine that uses warmed herbal oils customized for each dosha type.

The massage techniques range from light strokes to more intense tissue manipulation, with the goals of increasing circulation, eliminating toxins, and reestablishing dosha balance.

Beyond mere physical relaxation, Ayurvedic massage offers mental and emotional rejuvenation. It works by calming the nervous system and encouraging the release of feel-good hormones like dopamine and serotonin, which help reduce stress, anxiety, and fatigue. Regular Abhyanga is also thought to support lymphatic drainage and detoxification processes, which strengthen the immune system and improve skin health.

The choice of oils and particular massage techniques is based on an individual's dosha constitution and current health needs. For example, Vata types benefit from warm, grounding oils like sesame to pacify their tendency towards dryness and instability, Pitta types may use cooling oils like coconut or sunflower to soothe inflammation and heat-related imbalances, and Kapha types benefit from stimulating oils like mustard or almond to invigorate circulation and reduce sluggishness.

Ayurvedic massage is also essential for preserving joint flexibility, muscle tone, and general vitality.

A deeper connection between mind, body, and spirit is fostered, and Ayurvedic massage integrates well with the body's natural healing mechanisms to promote holistic wellness. This is in line with Ayurveda's emphasis on preventive health practices and personalized care based on individual constitution and needs.

CHAPTER THREE

HOW TO BEGIN RECEIVING AYURVEDIC MASSAGE

SETTING UP YOUR AREA AND YOURSELF

To create a space that is conducive to healing and relaxation, it is important to prepare yourself and your space before beginning an Ayurvedic massage. To begin, locate a peaceful, quiet place where you won't be disturbed, such as a designated massage room or a quiet corner of your home. Remove any clutter from the area and make sure the temperature is comfortable, as warmth is especially beneficial for this kind of massage.

The next step is to mentally and physically prepare yourself. Spend a few minutes centering yourself through deep breathing or meditation. Decide on your goal for the massage, such as relaxation, rejuvenation, or addressing a particular health concern. This mental preparation helps you focus and amplifies the therapeutic benefits of the massage.

Make sure you have enough time allotted so you can slow down and enjoy the experience to the fullest.

Finally, collect anything you'll need nearby. This could include blankets, towels, and massage oils. Based on Ayurvedic principles, select oils that suit your body type or dosha (for example, Vata types should use sesame oil, Pitta types should use coconut oil, and Kapha types should use sunflower oil). Having everything ready ahead of time makes it easier to transition smoothly into the massage.

ESSENTIAL BASIC EQUIPMENT

While complex equipment is not necessary for Ayurvedic massage, a few basic items improve the experience and efficacy of the therapy. To begin, you'll need a stable, supportive surface for the recipient to lie on, like a massage table or padded mat on the floor, to encourage relaxation and avoid discomfort.

In addition, prepare a few soft towels or sheets that can be used to cover the person getting the massage for privacy and warmth; they can also be used to remove extra oil from the skin or support the person's joints throughout the massage.

For example, sesame oil is often used for Vata types because of its warming and grounding properties; coconut oil is cooling and soothing, perfect for Pitta types; sunflower oil is lighter and more appropriate for Kapha types, helping with detoxification and invigorating; and so on. Choosing the appropriate type of oil is important when it comes to Ayurvedic massage because different oils are recommended for different doshas (body types) to balance energies and enhance therapeutic effects.

Lastly, make sure you have everything you need to provide a smooth and enjoyable Ayurvedic massage experience by keeping a small bowl or container for your massage oil close by, along with any other tools you may use, like herbal compresses or aroma diffusers to set the mood.

THE ENVIRONMENT IS IMPORTANT FOR MASSAGE

An Ayurvedic massage's effectiveness and overall experience are greatly influenced by the setting in which it is performed.

A calm, harmonious environment promotes deep relaxation in the recipient and facilitates the full expression of the massage's therapeutic effects.

First things first: make sure the room is warm enough to comfortably relax muscles and enhance the absorption of the massage oils; lighten the space with gentle lighting, avoiding harsh overhead lights that can be uncomfortable or distracting; soft music (instrumental or natural) can further enhance relaxation and create a calming ambiance.

Clearing the physical space of clutter and distractions will help you and the recipient concentrate fully on the message without outside interference. You can use natural elements to purify the air and create a relaxing aroma that enhances the massage, such as fresh flowers, essential oils, or incense.

Ayurvedically speaking, the setting should ideally balance the energies (doshas) of the parties involved. This can be accomplished by using particular colors or scents that correspond to the dosha of the recipient, which will enhance the therapeutic effects of the massage. In summary, a well-thought-out setting enhances the physical benefits of the massage as well as promotes a deeper sense of well-being and relaxation.

HYGIENE AND SAFETY PROCEDURES

To ensure a positive and healthy experience, it is imperative to uphold safety and hygiene standards when giving or receiving an Ayurvedic massage.

To start, wash your hands thoroughly before starting the massage to prevent the transfer of bacteria or germs. This also goes for any tools or equipment you may use during the session.

If using towels or sheets make sure they are freshly cleaned and devoid of any harsh detergents or smells that could cause pain. Make sure the massage area is clean and free of allergens or irritants that could harm the recipient's skin or respiratory system.

When choosing massage oils, consider any allergies the recipient may have; patch test a tiny area of skin before using a large amount to be sure there are no negative responses.

Respect the recipient's personal space and modesty during the massage to establish a safe and courteous environment for both of you. Check-in with the recipient frequently to make sure they are comfortable and make any necessary adjustments to methods or pressure.

Give the recipient some time to recuperate and assimilate the therapeutic effects of the massage; offer water or herbal tea to hydrate and assist the body's natural detoxification processes; and clean and sterilize any equipment used in the massage to maintain hygienic standards for subsequent sessions.

Prioritizing safety and sanitary procedures helps to boost the recipient's general well-being and relaxation in addition to increasing the effectiveness of the Ayurvedic massage.

ESTABLISHING GOALS FOR THE MASSAGE

Intention-setting during an Ayurvedic massage session enhances the therapeutic benefits of the practice by guiding the mind, body, and spirit toward specific goals. Decide what you want the massage to accomplish, such as relaxation and decompression, physical tension release, or specific health issues like stress management or digestive problems.

If you're giving a massage to someone else, once you've made your intention clear, share it with them. This helps establish a common goal and comprehension of the session's objectives, which builds a stronger bond and trust between the giver and the recipient.

Next, create an environment that is supportive of your intention. This can be as simple as adjusting the lighting and temperature to further enhance the mood and comfort of the space choosing appropriate music or sounds that encourage relaxation or using aromatherapy oils that correspond with the recipient's dosha or desired outcomes.

Encourage the recipient to focus on their intention, provide guidance through breathing exercises or relaxation techniques if necessary, and maintain mindfulness throughout the massage. Whether you are giving or receiving the massage, after the session take a moment to consider how the experience matched the intention and express gratitude for the healing energy that was shared. This helps to confirm the benefits of intention-setting and promotes continued mindfulness in future Ayurvedic massage sessions.

CHAPTER FOUR
THE APPLICATIONS OF AYURVEDIC OILS
A SUMMARY OF VITAL AYURVEDIC OILS

The foundation of traditional healing practices is Ayurvedic oils, which are known for their holistic benefits and therapeutic properties. These oils are made from natural sources like herbs, flowers, and roots and are carefully prepared to harness their potent medicinal qualities. Each oil has specific therapeutic properties that address different health needs, from body rejuvenation to mind calming. For example, sesame, coconut, and almond oils are commonly used bases because of their nourishing and emollient qualities, which are ideal for promoting skin health and overall well-being.

Ayurvedic oil selection is based on both the oil's inherent qualities and the individual's doshic constitution. Warming oils, like sesame, help balance the airy nature of Vata types and help them ground.

Intense, hot, Pitta types find relief from cooling oils, like coconut or sunflower, which balance excess heat and soothe inflammation. Kapha types, who are prone to congestion and sluggishness, benefit from stimulating oils, like mustard or eucalyptus, which are known for their energizing and uplifted qualities.

Applied regularly through massage rituals, Ayurvedic oils improve skin texture, circulation, detoxification, and relaxation. Their holistic approach goes beyond physical benefits to encompass mental and emotional well-being, aligning with the principles of balance and harmony. Infused with herbs and spices that enhance their therapeutic effects, such as turmeric for its anti-inflammatory properties or neem for its purifying benefits, Ayurvedic oils penetrate deeply into the tissues, nourishing from within.

QUALITIES AND ADVANTAGES OF ESSENTIAL OILS

Ancient wisdom has led to the reverence for Ayurvedic oils, which are highly valued for their multifarious benefits that address both physical and mental well-being. Warming essential oils, such as sesame, work deep into tissues to relieve stiffness and encourage joint flexibility. Cooling oils, like coconut oil, calm inflammation and nourish sensitive skin, so Pitta types who are experiencing heat-related imbalances will find relief from these oils.

Medicinal herbs and botanical extracts are frequently added to Ayurvedic formulations to augment their therapeutic efficacy, going beyond their base oils. For example, ashwagandha-infused oils are highly valued for their adaptogenic qualities, which assist the body in managing stress and exhaustion while fostering resilience. Turmeric, with its strong anti-inflammatory and antioxidant characteristics, is frequently mixed with oils to promote joint health and general vitality.

Ayurvedic oils are not just useful for physical ailments; they also help with mental and emotional balance. Aromatherapy oils, such as lavender or jasmine, are highly valued for their calming properties and their capacity to relieve stress, anxiety, and insomnia. Using these oils in massage therapy regularly not only benefits the body but also balances the mind and promotes emotional fortitude and inner peace.

COMBINING OILS FOR VARIOUS DOSHAS

The art of blending oils in Ayurveda is governed by the principles of balancing the doshas (Vata, Pitta, and Kapha) to achieve the best possible health and well-being. Since each dosha has distinct qualities, blending oils effectively requires choosing base oils that balance the predominant doshic qualities and adding herbs and spices to enhance therapeutic benefits.

Warming oils like sesame or almond are mixed with grounding herbs like ashwagandha or Bala for the Vata dosha, which is characterized by cold, dry, and unpredictable features. These mixtures not only nourish the skin but also soothe the nervous system and encourage warmth and stability in the body.

Pitta dosha is characterized by heat and intensity; therefore, mixes of cooling oils, like coconut or sunflower, combined with calming herbs, like rose or sandalwood, work well to balance excess heat, calm inflammation and encourage a feeling of cooling and relaxation.

With its features of heaviness and congestion, the Kapha dosha thrives when energizing herbs like juniper or ginger are coupled with stimulating oils like mustard or eucalyptus. These combinations assist in awakening the senses, encourage circulation, and drive out stagnation, so bringing back vitality and energy.

SELECTING THE PROPER OIL BASED ON YOUR BODY TYPE

Ayurveda classifies people into three main body types, or doshas, each of which has unique physical, emotional, and psychological characteristics. The selection of oil is based on these innate qualities, which ensure that it harmonizes and complements the predominant doshic tendencies. Choosing the right Ayurvedic oil for your body type is crucial to optimizing therapeutic benefits and preserving domestic balance.

Warming oils like sesame, almond, or jojoba are very helpful for Vata types, who are prone to dryness, coldness, and erratic energy. These oils increase circulation, deep nourishment, and the nervous system, which helps to promote stability and anchoring.

Cooling oils like coconut, sunflower, or ghee are beneficial for Pitta types, who are hot, intense, and have a high metabolism. They reduce inflammation, balance heat, and nourish sensitive skin, which helps to create a peaceful and relaxed feeling.

The heaviness, sluggishness, and congestion associated with the kapha type are best suited for stimulating oils such as juniper, eucalyptus, or mustard; they stimulate the senses, encourage circulation, assist break the cycle of stagnation and lethargy, and provide a revitalized sense of vitality.

Selecting the appropriate oil requires knowledge of your doshic constitution to choose oils that balance out any imbalances or discomforts related to your dominant dosha. Using these oils regularly in massage rituals promotes general health and well-being in line with Ayurvedic principles while also nurturing the skin.

TECHNIQUES FOR USING OIL IN MASSAGE

Ayurvedic massage oil application is a healing modality that combines physical, emotional, and spiritual aspects of well-being. The techniques used in oil application are intended to improve absorption, encourage relaxation, and balance the doshas, which maintains a balanced flow of energy throughout the body.

Abhyanga is one of the main techniques: warm oil is applied methodically in gentle circular motions to massage the entire body; this ritual not only nourishes the skin but also stimulates lymphatic drainage, detoxifies the body, and encourages deep relaxation of the nervous system and muscles.

Shirodhara is another technique that targets the Third Eye (Ajna) chakra by continuously applying warm oil to the forehead; it is especially beneficial for anxiety, insomnia, and neurological disorders because it calms the mind, reduces stress, and improves mental clarity and focus.

Localized therapies apply oils directly to body parts that are tense, painful, or imbalanced; these targeted massages use pressure, friction, and kneading techniques to release knots in the muscles, increase blood flow, and reduce discomfort.

Whether applied through full-body massages or targeted treatments, the principles of Ayurvedic oil application promote harmony and balance within the body-mind complex.

CHAPTER FIVE
AYURVEDIC MASSAGE METHODS
ABHYANGA: CONVENTIONAL METHOD OF SELF-MASSAGE

Abhyanga is a foundational practice in Ayurveda, known for its therapeutic benefits and ability to promote overall well-being. This traditional self-massage technique involves using warm oils, typically infused with herbs tailored to one's dosha, to nourish the skin, relax muscles, and balance the mind.

To begin, warm the massage oil slightly to a comfortable temperature, ensuring it's not too hot. Start with the scalp, using gentle circular motions to stimulate circulation and release tension. Gradually move to the face, ears, neck, and shoulders, using long strokes along the limbs and circular motions on joints to improve flexibility and joint health. Abhyanga isn't just about physical benefits; it's also a meditative practice that fosters a deeper connection between mind, body, and spirit.

Regular practice of Abhyanga promotes relaxation, supports lymphatic drainage, enhances skin texture, and balances the doshas. Integrating this self-care ritual into your routine can bring profound benefits to your overall health and well-being.

VARIOUS STROKES AND THEIR OBJECTIVES

The specific purposes of the strokes used in Ayurvedic massage are to balance the body's energy flow and doshic balance; long, relaxing strokes help distribute the oil evenly and calm the nervous system; circular motions around joints and tension areas release blockages and improve joint mobility; kneading and tapping movements stimulate circulation and detoxification; the pressure used varies: lighter for sensitive areas and deeper for areas that need to release tension and stagnation; knowing these techniques helps customize the massage to each individual's needs, ensuring maximum therapeutic benefit; each stroke works to promote balance, rejuvenation, and harmony within the body's subtle energy systems, supporting general health and vitality.

IN AN AYURVEDIC MASSAGE, MARMA POINTS

Marma points are vital energy centers located throughout the body where muscles, joints, veins, arteries, tendons, bones, and tissues intersect. In Ayurvedic massage, stimulating these points helps clear energy blockages, enhance prana (life force), and promote healing. Each marma point corresponds to different bodily functions and organs, influencing both physical and energetic systems. For example, pressing gently on the marma point associated with the heart can relieve emotional stress and support cardiac health. Understanding and correctly applying marma point therapy requires knowledge of their locations and functions. Integrating marma point stimulation into an Ayurvedic massage enhances its therapeutic benefits, promoting deep relaxation, balancing the doshas, and supporting overall well-being.

By learning to identify and stimulate these points effectively, practitioners can offer a profound healing experience that aligns with the principles of Ayurveda, promoting holistic health and vitality.

CHANGING PRESSURE BASED ON DOSHA

Understanding these doshic differences allows practitioners to tailor the massage experience, ensuring it addresses specific imbalances and promotes harmony within the body. By adjusting pressure and oil selection according to the client's dosha, Ayurvedic massage becomes a personalized therapy that supports overall health and well-being. Vata types benefit from gentle, warming strokes to calm their nervous system and ground their energy; Pitta types respond well to cooling strokes that reduce inflammation and promote relaxation; and Kapha types benefit from stimulating, invigorating strokes to enhance circulation and uplift their energy.

INCLUDING AWARENESS OF BREATH

Incorporating deep, mindful breathing into the massage practice helps release tension, improve the oxygenation of tissues, and support detoxification processes. By synchronizing breath with massage movements, practitioners can create a holistic healing experience that integrates body, mind, and spirit. Breath awareness is essential to Ayurvedic massage because it enhances the therapeutic effects by calming the mind, promoting relaxation, and facilitating energy flow. Additionally, encouraging clients to focus on their breath during the massage helps deepen their relaxation response and enhances the body's ability to absorb the healing benefits of the oils and strokes.

CHAPTER SIX

AYURVEDIC MASSAGE BENEFITS

PHYSICAL ADVANTAGES: CIRCULATION, MUSCLE RELAXATION, AND JOINT HEALTH

For starters, Ayurvedic massage has a great deal to offer in terms of physical benefits. Using firm but gentle strokes and specific herbal oils, the massage promotes lubrication of joints, increasing flexibility and decreasing stiffness. This helps to maintain joint mobility and prevent conditions like arthritis. Moreover, the techniques target muscle relaxation by relieving tense muscles and releasing built-up tension, which not only relieves immediate discomfort but also gradually improves overall muscle tone and flexibility.

Improved circulation supports faster muscle recovery after physical exertion and enhances overall vitality. This holistic approach to physical well-being through Ayurvedic massage ensures that both joints and muscles benefit, promoting long-term health and mobility. Additionally, Ayurvedic massage stimulates circulation throughout the body. The rhythmic motions and pressure applied during the massage encourage blood flow.

BENEFITS FOR THE MIND: REDUCTION OF STRESS AND EMOTIONAL HARMONY

Stress relief is the most common benefit that Ayurvedic massage is known for. The techniques employed in this age-old practice help to calm the nervous system, reducing levels of stress hormones like cortisol. The mind experiences a deep sense of relaxation and tranquility as the body relaxes under the expert hands and aromatic oils. This relaxation response not only alleviates stress symptoms but also promotes mental clarity and emotional balance.

Additionally, by harmonizing the body's energy centers, or chakras, Ayurvedic massage promotes emotional balance. By opening up blocked energy and bringing these centers back into balance, the massage helps people feel more emotionally resilient and stable. This emotional stability can help manage mood swings, anxiety, and depression, which can help people have a more positive outlook on life. With regular practice, Ayurvedic massage becomes an essential tool for maintaining mental well-being and improving overall emotional health.

EFFECTS OF DETOXIFICATION AND CLEANING

Ayurveda emphasizes the importance of eliminating toxins, or ama, from the body to maintain health and prevent disease. Ayurvedic massage techniques, combined with therapeutic oils specifically chosen for their detoxifying properties, facilitate the elimination of toxins through the skin, lymphatic system, and other eliminatory channels. This is one of the main benefits of Ayurvedic massage: its profound detoxification and cleansing effects on the body.

Regular sessions of Ayurvedic massage help people feel more energized, their skin clearer, and their overall vitality increased.

The massage strokes and herbal oils used in Ayurvedic massage stimulate the lymphatic system, which is important for detoxification. This helps to flush out accumulated toxins and waste products from the body's tissues, promoting cellular health and rejuvenation.

Additionally, the gentle kneading and friction techniques used during the massage enhance circulation, further supporting the body's natural detoxification processes.

BOOSTING VITALITY AND IMMUNITY

Improved lymphatic circulation aids in strengthening the immune response, making the body more resilient against infections and illnesses. Ayurvedic massage greatly contributes to enhancing immunity and vitality by supporting the body's natural defense mechanisms. The massage techniques stimulate the flow of lymph, a key component of the immune system, which helps in identifying and fighting off pathogens.

In addition, Ayurvedic massage enhances overall vitality and resilience by balancing the body's doshas, or biological energies. Restoring harmony between the Vata, Pitta, and Kapha doshas addresses imbalances, and the balanced state not only supports mental clarity and emotional well-being but also boosts physical stamina. Regular practice of Ayurvedic massage thus becomes a proactive approach to maintaining optimal health and vitality throughout life.

BENEFITS OF REGULAR PRACTICE OVER TIME

Frequent Ayurvedic massage therapy has long-term advantages for mental and physical health, promoting holistic health. In terms of physical benefits, regular massage therapy sessions lead to increased joint flexibility, decreased muscle tension, and improved circulation, which not only ease present discomfort but also prevent future musculoskeletal problems, promoting overall mobility and longevity.

When Ayurvedic massage is incorporated into a person's wellness routine, they experience a constant state of relaxation and emotional resilience. This proactive approach to mental health supports cognitive function, emotional stability, and overall quality of life. The cumulative effects of Ayurvedic massage on the mind include sustained stress relief, emotional balance, and heightened mental clarity.

Furthermore, the detoxifying and immune-boosting properties of Ayurvedic massage guarantee continuous cleansing and revitalization of the body's systems. By consistently getting rid of toxins and boosting immunity, Ayurvedic massage contributes to long-term robust health and vitality. In the end, the long-term advantages of Ayurvedic massage emphasize its function as a holistic therapeutic approach for fostering long-lasting physical, mental, and emotional well-being.

CHAPTER SEVEN

TAILORING YOUR PRACTICE TO AYURVEDIC MASSAGE

MASSAGING DEPENDING ON THE SEASON (RITUCHARYA)

Since each season corresponds to a different dosha (Vata, Pitta, and Kapha) that influences our physical and mental states, in Ayurveda, adjusting your massage practice to the seasons (Ritucharya) is crucial to keeping your body and mind in balance and harmony all year long. For example, in the cold, dry Vata season (fall and early winter), warming and nourishing oils like sesame or almond infused with warming herbs like ginger or cinnamon are recommended. These oils help to counterbalance Vata's tendency towards dryness and instability, promoting grounding and relaxation.

In the moist, cool Kapha season (late winter and spring), stimulating oils like mustard or eucalyptus, infused with invigorating herbs like cloves or juniper, help to energize and uplift. These oils can counteract Kapha's tendency towards sluggishness and congestion, promoting vitality and clarity. As the season shifts to the hot, intense Pitta period (summer), cooling oils like coconut or sunflower, infused with calming herbs like rose or sandalwood, can pacify Pitta's fiery nature.

Ritucharya promotes mindfulness and adaptation, which makes it easy to harmonize with seasonal changes. By modifying your massage oils and techniques according to each season, you may connect with nature's rhythms and assist your body's intrinsic healing processes.

MODIFYING METHODS CONSIDERING AGE AND CONSTITUTION

To maximize the benefits of massage therapy, it is important to modify Ayurvedic massage techniques according to age and individual constitution (Prakriti). Vata, Pitta, and Kapha are the three main constitutions (doshas) recognized by Ayurveda; each has distinct qualities that influence physical, mental, and emotional traits. Vata types are generally creative and energetic, but they can also be prone to anxiety and dry skin. Pitta types are usually driven and focused, but they can also be prone to inflammation and stress. Finally, Kapha types are often calm and stable, but they may also struggle with sluggishness and congestion.

The energy levels and physical sensitivities of young children and elderly people differ, so gentler massage techniques and softer oils are needed. For children, calming herbs like lavender or chamomile infused with light, nourishing oils like almond or coconut can support healthy growth and relaxation. For the elderly, warm, grounding oils like sesame or olive infused with rejuvenating herbs like ashwagandha or ginseng can help relieve stiffness and increase circulation.

When using Ayurvedic massage techniques, age and constitution are taken into account, so you can successfully customize the therapy to meet each person's demands. This individualized approach boosts the therapeutic advantages of massage, supporting longevity and general well-being.

TAKING CARE OF PARTICULAR HEALTH ISSUES

Targeting imbalances in the body and mind, Ayurvedic massage offers a comprehensive approach to treating specific health concerns. Whether treating digestive problems, stress-related disorders, or chronic pain, Ayurvedic principles direct practitioners to choose the right oils, herbs, and techniques to relieve symptoms and restore equilibrium. For example, people with chronic pain may find that warming oils like sesame or mustard, when paired with pain-relieving herbs like turmeric or ginger, help to reduce inflammation and facilitate healing.

Digestive disorders like bloating or indigestion can be effectively treated with digestive oils like fennel or peppermint, which aid in digestion and reduce discomfort. Calming oils like coconut or sandalwood, infused with relaxing herbs like brahmi or jatamansi, can help to induce a sense of calmness and tranquility, balancing the nervous system and promoting restful sleep.

People can receive profound healing benefits on a physical, mental, and emotional level by incorporating Ayurvedic massage into a comprehensive treatment plan that is customized to address specific health concerns. This integrative approach supports the body's natural healing mechanisms and promotes holistic well-being.

INCLUDING AYURVEDIC PRINCIPLES IN EVERYDAY LIVING

Ayurveda emphasizes daily self-care practices, known as Dinacharya, which include rituals like oil pulling, tongue scraping, and self-massage (Abhyanga) using therapeutic oils. Including these practices helps to cleanse the body of toxins (ama), enhance circulation, and promote overall vitality.

Applying Ayurvedic principles to daily life goes beyond the massage table, strengthening balance and harmony in everyday routines.

Daily self-massage not only nourishes the skin but also calms the mind, reduces stress, and enhances relaxation. Depending on your dosha type and current imbalances, you can choose the right oils and herbs for self-massage. Vata types may benefit from warming oils like sesame or almond, while Pitta types may prefer cooling oils like coconut or sunflower. Kapha types can benefit from stimulating oils like mustard or eucalyptus to invigorate and uplift.

To maintain optimal health and well-being, Ayurveda also recommends self-massage, mindful eating, adequate rest, regular exercise, and proper hydration. By incorporating Ayurvedic principles into your daily routine, you can develop a deeper connection with your body and environment, which will naturally promote longevity and vitality.

MASSAGE TECHNIQUES FOR FAMILIES AND PARTNERS

Ayurvedic massage goes beyond self-care for individuals to include partner and family practices, creating stronger bonds and enhancing mutual well-being. Partner massage makes it possible for people to support each other's health goals by addressing specific issues like stress relief or muscle tension, as well as bonding through nurturing touch, intimacy, and relaxation.

Effective communication and mutual respect are key components of partner massage. To start, choose appropriate oils according to each partner's dosha and preferences. For instance, if one partner is Pitta-dominant and the other is Vata-dominant, choose oils like sesame that balance both energies, as well as calming herbs like lavender or sandalwood. This will balance the massage and guarantee that both partners experience the therapeutic benefits of the massage.

Family members can take turns giving massages, creating a nurturing environment where everyone feels cared for and valued. Parents can introduce children to gentle massage techniques using safe, nourishing oils suitable for their age and constitution. Family massage practices can also promote harmony and well-being within the household.

It is possible to improve physical health as well as emotional and social bonds within the family by implementing partner and family massage practices into your routine. Ayurvedic massage becomes a shared experience of rejuvenation and relaxation, promoting overall wellness for all parties involved.

CHAPTER EIGHT
AYURVEDIC PRACTICES FOR SELF-CARE

DAILY ROUTINES FOR AYURVEDIC SELF-CARE

Ayurveda believes that self-care daily, or Dinacharya, is the cornerstone to preserving health and equilibrium. These practices include a series of rituals that are intended to harmonize with natural cycles and enhance general well-being. For example, part of a typical morning routine entails rising early to coincide with the body's natural energy cycles, scraping the tongue to eliminate toxins that have accumulated during the night, and oil pulling to improve oral hygiene and detoxification. Next, self-massaging with warm oil, or Abhyanga, is performed to nourish the skin, improve circulation, and soothe the nervous system. This practice is not only beneficial to the body; it also fosters a sense of groundedness and self-awareness.

Ayurvedic self-care throughout the day focuses on mindful eating and drinking plenty of water. Warm, freshly cooked meals eaten at regular intervals support digestion and assimilation of nutrients. Adding herbal teas or warm water with herbs like ginger or cumin aids in detoxification and maintains digestive fire. A brief meditation or breathing exercises to relieve stress and improve mental clarity are part of an afternoon self-care routine. Evening activities involve winding down, including light yoga stretches to relax the body and set the stage for sound sleep. Modest foot massages before bed encourage relaxation and assist in grounding excess energy accumulated during the day.

Ayurvedic self-care is all about being consistent. By progressively incorporating these practices into daily life, one can develop a stronger sense of self and support holistic health from the inside out.

ROUTINES ARE IMPORTANT (DINACHARYA)

In Ayurveda, the daily routine, or dinacharya, is very important for preserving equilibrium and enhancing general health. These routines are customized to individual constitutions (doshas) and seasonal variations to align with natural rhythms. Maintaining a regular daily routine supports the body's inherent detoxification processes and strengthens resistance to daily stressors.

For example, rising early in the morning is in line with the Vata time of day, which promotes alertness and vitality. Activities such as oil massage and nasal cleansing (Neti) aid in the removal of accumulated toxins and preserve sensory clarity.

Moreover, Dinacharya instills a sense of discipline and mindfulness, motivating people to prioritize self-care as an essential part of their daily lives. Regularity of routines also helps to regulate biological functions, such as digestion, sleep, and elimination.

Eating meals at regular times supports digestive fire (Agni), ensuring efficient nutrient absorption and waste elimination. Aligning daily activities with the sun's natural cycle helps to optimize energy levels throughout the day.

Ayurveda places a strong focus on routines, but they also apply to mental and emotional health. Through the creation and maintenance of personalized daily routines, individuals can develop resilience, inner harmony, and general vitality.

AYURVEDIC FOOD RECOMMENDATIONS FOR OPTIMAL HEALTH AND WELLNESS

Eating fresh, seasonal foods that are locally sourced and prepared mindfully is the foundation of Ayurvedic dietary guidelines, which are based on the principle of maintaining balance within the body and mind. At the heart of these guidelines is the concept of six tastes (Rasas) - sweet, sour, salty, bitter, pungent, and astringent - which should be included in meals to satisfy all aspects of the palate and promote digestion. Meals are ideally cooked fresh and eaten warm to support Agni (digestive fire) and ensure optimal nutrient absorption.

Eating by one's dominant dosha (Vata, Pitta, or Kapha) and the present state of balance or imbalance is another important Ayurvedic dietary practice. For instance, Vata types benefit from cooling foods like fresh fruits, leafy greens, and mild spices to balance their fiery nature; Pitta types benefit from light, stimulating foods like legumes, bitter greens, and pungent spices to counteract heaviness and sluggishness.

Ayurvedic dietary guidelines thus promote not only physical health but also a harmonious relationship between food, body, and mind. Apart from what is eaten, Ayurvedic practices like mindful eating, chewing food thoroughly, and eating in a calm, pleasant environment all enhance digestion and absorption of nutrients.

USING SPICES AND HERBS TO MAINTAIN BALANCE

Ayurvedic practice is replete with the use of herbs and spices, which are prized for their therapeutic qualities in preserving equilibrium and bolstering general health. Each herb and spice has unique effects that can affect the body's doshas (Vata, Pitta, and Kapha), fostering recovery and averting disease. For example, ginger is well known for its warming qualities, assisting in digestion, and relieving cold and congestion symptoms. Turmeric, on the other hand, is known for its anti-inflammatory and antioxidant qualities, which boost the immune system and joint health.

Herbs and spices are frequently used in Ayurvedic cooking, herbal teas, and medicinal preparations to address particular health issues or imbalances. For instance, Triphala, a blend of three fruits, is used to support regular bowel movements and detoxify the digestive system; ashwagandha, an adaptogen, offers stress relief and vitality; and cumin and coriander seeds are used in cooking to improve digestion and lessen gas and bloating.

Incorporating these natural remedies into daily life can support vitality, resilience, and balance, in line with the body's innate healing intelligence. Ayurvedic herb and spice selection and combination are governed by the principles of taste, potency, and therapeutic action, ensuring a holistic approach to health and well-being.

MASSAGE IN CONJUNCTION WITH YOGA AND MEDITATION

To maximize the therapeutic benefits of Ayurvedic massage, or Abhyanga, and support holistic well-being, yoga, and meditation practices are also recommended. Abhyanga is an Ayurvedic massage technique in which warm oil infused with herbs is applied to the skin and massaged into the skin to nourish tissues, improve circulation, and calm the nervous system.

This ritual not only promotes mental clarity and emotional balance but also enhances physical relaxation.

Yoga poses like Child's Pose and Cobra Pose help release tension from specific areas of the body, making it more receptive to massage. Pranayama techniques like Alternate Nostril Breathing (Nadi Shodhana) promote relaxation and enhance the flow of prana (life force) throughout the body. These practices can be integrated before or after Abhyanga to prepare the body and mind for massage and deepen its effects.

A deeper sense of relaxation and rejuvenation can be achieved by combining mindfulness meditation techniques (such as focusing on the breath or repeating a mantra) with Abhyanga or before it. This creates a synergistic effect that supports the body's natural healing processes and further promotes relaxation and mental clarity, complementing the physical benefits of massage.

CHAPTER NINE
FAQS & FREQUENTLY ASKED QUESTIONS

INTOLERANCES AND HYPERSENSITIVITY TO OILS

Allergies and oil sensitivity should be taken into account when receiving an Ayurvedic massage, as they can greatly affect the efficacy and safety of the massage. Many Ayurvedic oils come from natural sources, like sesame, coconut, or almond oils, and each offers special therapeutic benefits that are in line with Ayurvedic principles; however, people who are allergic to nuts should be cautious and choose oils that are safe for their particular sensitivities, like coconut oil, which is generally hypoallergenic. It is advisable to test a small amount of oil on a skin patch before applying it to the entire body to make sure there won't be any negative side effects.

Not only are oils used therapeutically in Ayurveda, but they are also chosen for their capacity to balance the body's doshas (Vata, Pitta, and Kapha). For instance, sesame oil is frequently used for its warming qualities, which are appropriate for balancing Vata dosha, while coconut oil's cooling qualities can pacify Pitta dosha. Knowledge of these properties aids in the selection of the appropriate oil for each individual, fostering relaxation as well as general well-being. It is always best to seek the advice of an Ayurvedic practitioner to determine the most appropriate oils based on your constitution and health condition to prevent allergic reactions or unfavorable effects during or after the massage.

To sum up, it is important to be aware of allergies and sensitivity to oils when receiving an Ayurvedic massage. By selecting oils carefully based on personal needs and speaking with a practitioner, one can benefit from Ayurveda's therapeutic benefits without worrying about allergic reactions. This approach guarantees a safe and efficient massage, which promotes both physical and emotional well-being.

PRECAUTIONARY MEASURES FOR EXPECTANT MOTHERS

Pregnancy can benefit greatly from Ayurvedic massage therapy, which relieves stress, improves circulation, and eases tense muscles. However, safety measures need to be taken to guarantee the health of the mother and unborn child during the massage. It is important to speak with a qualified Ayurvedic practitioner or healthcare provider before beginning any form of massage therapy during pregnancy. They can offer customized recommendations and guarantee that the massage techniques and oils used are safe and beneficial.

To minimize the risk of discomfort or harm, some pressure points and techniques should be avoided during pregnancy. For example, deep tissue massage and intense pressure on the abdomen should be avoided. Instead, gentle strokes and soothing techniques can be used to promote relaxation and ease common pregnancy-related discomforts. Finally, using safe pregnancy-safe oils, like coconut or sunflower oil, can further improve the massage experience without endangering the health of the mother or fetus.

In conclusion, when administered safely and under the supervision of a trained professional, Ayurvedic massage can be a beneficial component of prenatal care. Expectant mothers can reap the therapeutic benefits of Ayurveda while also protecting their health and the health of their unborn child by following the required safety protocols and using the right techniques and oils.

MODIFYING MASSAGE FOR OLDER OR ILL PEOPLE

Gentle strokes and light pressure can help alleviate muscle tension and improve circulation without causing discomfort or strain. Ayurvedic massage can be tailored to meet the specific needs of elderly or infirm individuals, offering gentle and comforting techniques that promote relaxation and improve overall well-being.

When working with elderly clients, it's important to consider their physical limitations, such as joint stiffness or frailty, and adjust the massage accordingly.

Ayurvedic principles emphasize the significance of customizing treatments to individual needs, ensuring that each session is both safe and beneficial. In addition, selecting warming and nourishing oils, like sesame or almond oil, can enhance the therapeutic effects of the massage for elderly individuals. These oils help lubricate the skin, reduce friction during massage, and promote a sense of warmth and comfort.

In summary, modifying Ayurvedic massage methods for older or disabled people entails applying light pressure, soft strokes, and appropriate oils to improve comfort and encourage relaxation. Taking into account the individual's particular physical circumstances and preferences, therapists can offer a restorative and revitalizing experience that promotes general health and well-being.

RESOLVING DOUBT REGARDING AYURVEDIC METHODS

Because of cultural differences, unfamiliarity, or misconceptions regarding their efficacy, Ayurvedic practices—including massage therapy—can occasionally be met with skepticism. Nevertheless, by comprehending the fundamentals and advantages of Ayurveda, one can counter these worries and underscore the system's significance as a holistic healthcare provider. Ayurveda stresses an individual's personalized approach to wellness, accounting for their particular constitution, lifestyle, and surroundings.

One prevalent misperception is that Ayurvedic treatments are wholly alternative and unsupported by science; in actuality, contemporary research is beginning to validate many Ayurvedic principles and practices, including the application of herbal medicines and therapeutic massage for a wide range of health conditions. Therapeutic massage, for example, is acknowledged for its capacity to enhance relaxation, balance the body's energies (doshas), improve circulation, and enhance general well-being.

To sum up, dispelling doubts about Ayurvedic practices requires educating people about its tenets, and advantages, and expanding the body of scientific evidence.

By highlighting Ayurveda's holistic approach to health and customized wellness plans, people can recognize Ayurveda as a useful adjunct to traditional medicine, providing significant therapeutic benefits for both the prevention and treatment of a wide range of illnesses.

HOW OFTEN IS AN AYURVEDIC MASSAGE RECOMMENDED?

Ayurvedic practitioners generally recommend regular massage sessions to maintain balance and promote overall well-being. If an individual has specific health conditions, bi-weekly or monthly sessions may be more beneficial than weekly ones. The frequency of Ayurvedic massage sessions depends on the individual's health goals, constitution (dosha balance), and specific health conditions.

Seasonal variations and lifestyle variables can also affect how frequently an Ayurvedic massage is administered. In times of stress or seasonal shift, the body may benefit from more frequent massages to support adaptation and resilience; in times of stability and good health, fewer sessions may be necessary to sustain optimal well-being.

An Ayurvedic practitioner can offer customized recommendations to maximize the therapeutic benefits of massage therapy, promoting both physical rejuvenation and emotional balance. The frequency of Ayurvedic massage should be customized based on individual needs, health goals, and lifestyle factors.

CHAPTER TEN

IMPROVING YOUR WORK

ADVANCED AYURVEDIC METHODS AND TREATMENTS

Ayurveda, an ancient Indian medical system, offers profound insights into personalized wellness through therapies like Panchakarma, a detoxification process aimed at cleansing the body of toxins accumulated over time. Panchakarma involves a series of treatments, including herbal massages, steam baths, and internal cleansing procedures tailored to individual dosha imbalances—Vata, Pitta, and Kapha. By addressing advanced techniques and therapies, one can delve into the rich tapestry of holistic healing practices that have developed over centuries.

In addition, Ayurvedic treatments like Abhyanga, or oil massage, are essential for fostering both physical and mental health. Abhyanga is a therapeutic massage that is applied to the body using warm herbal oils infused with healing botanicals. It is a cornerstone of Ayurvedic self-care practices because it relaxes the body and calms the mind. Marma therapy, on the other hand, targets specific energy points in the body and uses light pressure to release blockages and stimulate the flow of prana, or life force, promoting general vitality and emotional equilibrium.

Advanced Ayurvedic techniques are deeply beneficial when practiced under expert supervision; they support the body's natural healing processes and foster a harmonious relationship between mind, body, and spirit. However, incorporating these techniques into one's wellness routine requires understanding one's constitution and imbalances, seeking guidance from experienced practitioners, and respecting the holistic approach that integrates physical, mental, and spiritual dimensions of health.

RESOURCES AND ONGOING EDUCATION

Ayurveda, which is based on a holistic approach to health, offers a variety of avenues for ongoing learning, including specialized courses, workshops, and accredited programs that delve into the principles and applications of this venerable medical science. These educational opportunities not only provide theoretical knowledge but also emphasize practical skills, like herbal formulation, pulse diagnosis, and therapeutic techniques like Shirodhara, which involves pouring warm herbal oils on the forehead to induce deep relaxation and balance. Continuing education in Ayurveda is therefore imperative for practitioners and enthusiasts alike who wish to expand their knowledge and hone their skills in this age-old healing art.

There are many resources available for learning about Ayurveda. These include classic texts such as the Sushruta Samhita and Charaka Samhita, as well as contemporary interpretations and clinical studies that confirm Ayurveda's effectiveness in treating a range of health conditions. Online platforms and educational institutions also provide extensive curricula that are appropriate for learners of all skill levels, from novices to experts. Finally, continuing education cultivates a community of practitioners dedicated to maintaining and advancing Ayurvedic knowledge, guaranteeing its applicability in modern healthcare settings.

When someone starts an Ayurvedic journey, having access to trustworthy resources and ongoing education guarantees that they have a comprehensive understanding of this holistic science. By staying up to date on new research, evolving practices, and applying Ayurvedic principles to everyday life, practitioners can develop a greater understanding of the interdependence of health and well-being as promoted by the age-old wisdom of Ayurveda.

LOCATING ELIGIBLE AYURVEDIC PHYSICIANS

Discovering qualified Ayurvedic practitioners means sifting through a landscape full of diversity and tradition to make sure that practitioners have the education, training, and experience needed to provide genuine Ayurvedic care. Ayurveda is known throughout the world for its holistic approach to health and emphasizes the value of individualized consultations and treatments based on each patient's unique constitution and imbalances. Qualified practitioners frequently go through extensive training in Ayurvedic principles, diagnosis techniques, and therapeutic modalities.

To find respectable Ayurvedic doctors, people can get recommendations from reliable sources like medical doctors, integrative medicine wellness centers, or Ayurvedic associations that maintain high standards of practice and moral behavior. It is important to confirm credentials, such as educational background, certifications, and membership in reputable Ayurvedic associations or institutions. A licensed doctor will perform a full examination, including pulse diagnosis (Nadi Pariksha) and a thorough history-taking, to identify the underlying cause of health issues and prescribe customized treatments that are in line with Ayurvedic principles.

Selecting a certified Ayurvedic practitioner entails building a cooperative relationship that is founded on mutual respect, trust, and understanding of Ayurveda's holistic approach to health and well-being. By placing a high value on practitioner credentials, ethical compliance, and a dedication to continuous professional growth, people can set out on a path of self-healing and Ayurvedic wisdom.

INCLUDING THE PHILOSOPHY OF AYURVEDA IN DAILY LIFE

Ayurveda, which originated from ancient Indian wisdom, emphasizes harmony between mind, body, and spirit through personalized lifestyle practices, dietetics, and daily routines. Central to Ayurvedic philosophy is the concept of doshas—Vata, Pitta, and Kapha—which govern physiological functions and influence individual preferences, tendencies, and vulnerabilities. Integrating Ayurvedic philosophy into daily life encourages people to embrace a holistic approach to health and well-being that aligns with natural rhythms and individual constitutions.

Ayurvedic teachings encourage mindful eating practices, emphasizing the importance of fresh, seasonal foods that support digestion and nourish body tissues according to individual needs. Practical applications of Ayurvedic philosophy include following a daily routine (Dinacharya) tailored to one's predominant dosha and seasonal variations, incorporating specific dietary guidelines to balance dosha imbalances, and practicing mindfulness techniques like meditation and yoga to promote mental clarity and emotional resilience.

Ayurveda offers useful tools for fostering balance, vitality, and inner harmony amidst the demands of modern living. Whether through self-care rituals, mindful movement, or conscious food choices, individuals can cultivate practices that promote optimal health and well-being and a deeper awareness of their unique constitution by incorporating Ayurvedic principles into their daily lives.

EXAMINING WORKSHOPS & RETREATS FOR AYURVEDIC WELLNESS

Ayurvedic retreats are designed to immerse participants in holistic therapies, including daily yoga sessions, meditation practices, Ayurvedic massages, and individualized consultations with experienced practitioners. These retreats often take place in serene natural settings conducive to healing and relaxation, allowing participants to disconnect from daily stressors and reconnect with their inner selves. Learning about Ayurvedic wellness retreats and workshops offers an immersive experience of the principles and practices of this ancient healing tradition, providing opportunities for rejuvenation, self-discovery, and personal transformation.

Ayurvedic workshops introduce participants to fundamental ideas like dosha theory, Ayurvedic nutrition, herbal medicine, and lifestyle practices based on individual constitutions. Skilled instructors and practitioners lead participants through practical learning experiences, enabling them to incorporate

Ayurvedic wisdom into their lives for improved well-being. Retreats and workshops also provide a platform for community building, bringing like-minded people who are dedicated to holistic health and personal development together.

Whether you're looking for relaxation, rejuvenation, or deeper self-awareness, Ayurvedic wellness retreats and workshops offer a transformative journey rooted in holistic healing and harmony. By giving participants practical tools and insights to cultivate balance, vitality, and resilience in their lives, they can inspire profound shifts in health and perspective.

CHAPTER ELEVEN
UPCOMING DEVELOPMENTS IN AYURVEDIC MASSAGE

CONTEMPORARY USES AND INNOVATIONS

With roots in ancient Indian tradition, Ayurvedic massage has found new life in modern applications and innovations. Practitioners now combine age-old wisdom with cutting-edge methods and tools to improve therapeutic results. Innovations include the use of customized oils and herbal formulations based on each client's unique constitution (dosha), which promotes targeted healing in addition to relaxation. Modern methods prioritize client comfort and hygiene while maintaining Ayurvedic principles of balance and holistic wellness.

New techniques go beyond technique to include customized wellness programs that combine diet, lifestyle modifications, and mindfulness exercises. These integrative regimens target mental and emotional health issues in addition to physical illnesses, meeting the increasing need for natural and integrative healthcare options. Research has supported these innovations by confirming the validity of Ayurvedic principles and broadening the conditions for which Ayurvedic massage is advised.

Ayurvedic massage therapists now work in tandem with other healthcare professionals to promote integrative models that integrate Western medicine and complementary therapies with Ayurveda, improving treatment efficacy while expanding access to Ayurvedic practices worldwide. With the growing recognition of the advantages of holistic care in contemporary healthcare systems, Ayurvedic massage has become an essential part of wellness programs designed to fend off illness and encourage longevity.

GROWING WORLDWIDE ADOPTION OF AYURVEDIC PRACTICES

Based on ancient Indian wisdom, Ayurveda's holistic approach appeals to a diverse audience looking for personalized health solutions.

The surge in popularity is driven by growing awareness of Ayurvedic principles, which emphasize the balance of mind, body, and spirit through lifestyle adjustments, herbal remedies, and therapeutic practices like massage. Ayurvedic massage is one of the many natural alternatives to conventional medicine that people are turning to.

Around the world, Ayurvedic spas and wellness centers provide a variety of treatments, bringing these age-old therapies within reach of a growing number of people. Ayurvedic massage schools have sprung up in response to this demand, guaranteeing a new wave of practitioners skilled in providing genuine, high-quality treatments. This growth has been bolstered by studies that demonstrate the effectiveness of Ayurvedic therapies in treating chronic illnesses, boosting immunity, and fostering general health.

The global community continues to embrace and incorporate Ayurvedic principles into modern lifestyles as governments and healthcare institutions respond to increased demand by incorporating Ayurvedic practices into public health initiatives, realizing their potential to supplement conventional medicine. This mainstream acceptance highlights Ayurveda's role not just as a complementary therapy but as a cornerstone of preventive healthcare.

INTEGRATIVE METHODS IN MEDICAL PRACTICE

Integrative medicine unites Ayurveda with conventional medical practices, acknowledging the complementary benefits of both. This approach encourages collaboration between Ayurvedic practitioners, allopathic doctors, and specialists, ensuring comprehensive care that addresses the underlying causes of health issues.

Ayurvedic massage is becoming more and more integrated into contemporary healthcare frameworks, reflecting a broader shift towards holistic and patient-centered approaches.

Ayurvedic massage plays a crucial role in these models by promoting relaxation, reducing stress, and supporting the body's natural healing processes. Therapists tailor treatments based on individual dosha profiles and health concerns, ensuring personalized care that aligns with Ayurvedic principles of balance and harmony. Integrative healthcare models prioritize patient education and empowerment, encouraging individuals to take an active role in their well-being.

As integrative therapies gain more traction, research confirms that Ayurvedic massage is effective in treating ailments like anxiety, digestive disorders, and chronic pain. Ayurvedic massage is becoming more and more important in multidisciplinary treatment plans as healthcare systems transition to more holistic approaches that combine traditional knowledge with cutting-edge science to provide patients with all-encompassing care that puts long-term health and wellness first.

INVESTIGATIONS AND ADVANCEMENTS IN AYURVEDIC MEDICINE

Scientific studies validate the effectiveness of Ayurvedic principles in promoting health and treating various ailments. Ongoing research explores the biochemical mechanisms behind Ayurvedic treatments, shedding light on their physiological effects and potential applications in modern medicine. Research and development in Ayurvedic therapies, including massage, is driving innovation and enhancing therapeutic outcomes.

Research is also examining the neurobiological reactions to Ayurvedic oils and herbal formulations used in massage, uncovering their impact on neurotransmitter levels and stress hormones. These findings support the integration of Ayurvedic therapies into mainstream healthcare, expanding treatment options for patients worldwide. Clinical trials have demonstrated the benefits of Ayurvedic massage in improving circulation, reducing inflammation, and enhancing immune function.

Research is also being done on novel formulations and delivery systems to maximize the therapeutic effects of Ayurvedic massage. State-of-the-art methods of extracting herbs maintain their potency, and contemporary quality standards guarantee the safety and effectiveness of the products.

Research is also being done in collaboration with Ayurvedic practitioners, researchers, and pharmaceutical companies to create new therapies that fuse traditional knowledge with modern science.

NEW PROSPECTS FOR AYURVEDIC PROFESSIONALS

Increasing demand for Ayurvedic therapies, including massage, has created diverse career prospects in wellness centers, spas, hospitals, and private practice settings worldwide. Accredited training programs equip practitioners with the skills and knowledge needed to meet this demand, ensuring high standards of care and professionalism. Ayurvedic practitioners are well-positioned to take advantage of these emerging opportunities as interest in traditional healing practices continues to grow on a global scale.

Ayurvedic practitioners have many business options. They can open their clinics, consultancies, or product lines for health-conscious consumers. Adding Ayurvedic principles to mainstream healthcare systems opens up more opportunities for specialization and collaboration. Practitioners can collaborate with holistic therapists, allopathic physicians, and nutritionists to provide holistic health solutions that integrate Eastern and Western methods.

Technological developments in the fields of telemedicine and digital health also broaden the reach that Ayurvedic practitioners can have in reaching out to clients worldwide, enabling them to conduct virtual consultations and wellness programs. This digital revolution improves accessibility to Ayurvedic knowledge and treatments, which in turn creates a larger audience for traditional healing methods.

As Ayurveda becomes more widely accepted as a legitimate medical treatment, practitioners can anticipate further expansion and change in their professional lives, helping to further the field's global integrative medicine.

www.ingramcontent.com/pod-product-compliance
Lightning Source LLC
Chambersburg PA
CBHW071836210526
45479CB00001B/165